Epstein-Barr Virus

A Beginner's Step-by-Step Guide to Managing EBV Naturally Through Diet, With Sample Recipes and a Meal Plan

copyright © 2021 Jeffrey Winzant

All rights reserved No part of this book may be reproduced, or stored in a retrieval system, or transmitted in any form or by any means, electronic, mechanical, photocopying, recording, or otherwise, without express written permission of the publisher.

Disclaimer

By reading this disclaimer, you are accepting the terms of the disclaimer in full. If you disagree with this disclaimer, please do not read the guide.

All of the content within this guide is provided for informational and educational purposes only, and should not be accepted as independent medical or other professional advice. The author is not a doctor, physician, nurse, mental health provider, or registered nutritionist/dietician. Therefore, using and reading this guide does not establish any form of a physician-patient relationship.

Always consult with a physician or another qualified health provider with any issues or questions you might have regarding any sort of medical condition. Do not ever disregard any qualified professional medical advice or delay seeking that advice because of anything you have read in this guide. The information in this guide is not intended to be any sort of medical advice and should not be used in lieu of any medical advice by a licensed and qualified medical professional.

The information in this guide has been compiled from a variety of known sources. However, the author cannot attest to or guarantee the accuracy of each source and thus should not be held liable for any errors or omissions.

You acknowledge that the publisher of this guide will not be held liable for any loss or damage of any kind incurred as a result of this guide or the reliance on any information provided within this guide. You acknowledge and agree that you assume all risk and responsibility for any action you undertake in response to the information in this guide.

Using this guide does not guarantee any particular result (e.g., weight loss or a cure). By reading this guide, you acknowledge that there are no guarantees to any specific outcome or results you can expect.

All product names, diet plans, or names used in this guide are for identification purposes only and are the property of their respective owners. The use of these names does not imply endorsement. All other trademarks cited herein are the property of their respective owners.

Where applicable, this guide is not intended to be a substitute for the original work of this diet plan and is, at most, a supplement to the original work for this diet plan and never a direct substitute. This guide is a personal expression of the facts of that diet plan.

Where applicable, persons shown in the cover images are stock photography models and the publisher has obtained the rights to use the images through license agreements with third-party stock image companies.

Table of Contents

Introduction	7
What Is the Epstein-Barr Virus?	9
Recent Scientific Advances in Epstein-Barr Virus (EBV) Research	11
New Diagnostic Tools for Detecting Latent and Reactivated EBV	11
Emerging Therapies for EBV Management	13
Links Between EBV and Chronic Diseases	15
The EBV Stages	18
Stage One of Epstein-Barr	18
Stage Two of Epstein-Barr	20
Stage Three of Epstein-Barr Virus	22
Stage Four of Epstein-Barr Virus	23
How Epstein-Barr Virus (EBV) Affects Your Immune System	26
How EBV Impacts T-Cells and B-Cells	26
Chronic EBV and Weak Immune Defenses	27
How to Rebuild and Support Your Immune System	28
Health Complications Associated with EBV	31
Mental Health and EBV	32
Practical Stress Management Programs for EBV Recovery	37
How Chronic Stress Triggers EBV Reactivation	37
A 30-Day Mindfulness Challenge for EBV Recovery	37
Daily Breathing Exercises to Support Your Nervous System	39
Breaking the Cycle of Stress and EBV Reactivation	41
Natural Epstein-Barr Treatment Protocols	43
Transmission and Diagnosis	43
Natural Treatment for EBV Infections	46
Step 1: Drinking Plenty of Fluids	46
Step 2: Get Quality Restorative Rest	47
Step 3: Detoxify Your Body to Support The Immune System	47
Step 4: Moderate Exercises	53
Incorporating Herbal Remedies into Daily Life for EBV Management	55

    The Power of Herbs in EBV Management   55
    How to Incorporate Herbs Into Daily Life   56
    DIY Recipes for EBV-Supportive Herbs   58
    Dosage and Safety Precautions   60

Comprehensive Guide to Supplements for EBV Recovery   **62**
    Key Supplements for EBV Recovery   62
    The Role of Adaptogens in EBV Recovery   64
    Precautions for Combining Supplements with Medications   66

Customized Nutrition Plans for Different EBV Stages   **68**
    Stage 1: Latent Stage   68
    Stage 2: Active Stage   70
    Stage 3: Organ-Involved Stage   71
    Stage 4: Nervous System Stage   72

The Epstein-Barr Diet: Supporting Your Body with Nutrition   **75**
    EBV Healing Foods   76
    Foods to Avoid   78

Epstein-Barr Diet Plan and Sample Recipes   **80**
    Arugula and Mushroom Salad   81
    Avocado, Cucumber, and Tomato Salad   82
    Chicken Salad   83
    Egg Salad with Avocados   84
    Vegetable Broth   85
    Apricot-Glazed Salmon   87
    Salmon Salad   88
    Salmon with Avocados and Brussels Sprouts   89
    Blueberry-Banana Overnight Oats   92
    Salmon Soup   93
    Salad Medley   94

Conclusion   **96**
FAQs   **98**
References and Helpful Links   **101**

Introduction

If you have been diagnosed with Epstein-Barr Virus (EBV), you're not alone. EBV is one of the most common viral infections in humans. Around 90% of adults in the United States have been infected at some point in their lives, and most people don't even know it because the virus can be dormant for years.

Based on the many misconceptions surrounding this virus, it seems to be a fairly benign ailment. It is often referred to as "mono" or "the kissing disease" because it is so easily spread by physical contact with an infected person. However, the symptoms of this virus can be worse than anyone realizes and far more dangerous than people are led to believe.

But did you know that there are simple steps you can take to regain your health naturally?

From nutrition and supplements to lifestyle changes, the right approach can help you fight off EBV and leave you feeling better than you have in years. For more information on Epstein-Barr Virus, continue reading.

In this guide, you'll discover:

- The guiding principles of EBV management using natural methods
- The stages of the Epstein-Barr Virus
- EBV healing foods
- EBV healing herbs and food supplements
- How to diagnose and treat EBV infections
- Epstein-Barr diet sample recipes to follow

Keep reading to learn more about managing EBV naturally and regaining your health. By the end of this guide, you'll have a better understanding of how to combat this virus and live a healthier life.

What Is the Epstein-Barr Virus?

Epstein-Barr Virus, also known as EBV, is a ubiquitous human herpesvirus belonging to the herpesviridae family.

This type of virus has been linked to several immunologic and neurological disorders. It is also closely related to the herpes simplex viruses, and like other herpes viruses, EBV establishes lifelong infections in its host.

In recent studies, researchers concluded that EBV is the most common cause of infectious mononucleosis in up to 90% of adolescents and young adults in the US, usually causing symptoms that last for two to four weeks.

Here's where it gets tricky—many individuals have been infected with EBV in their lives without noticing, and they remain asymptomatic for decades. In contrast, the infection can cause symptoms in others when first infected with EBV.

Unlike the herpes simplex virus, EBV is said to be a double-stranded DNA virus.

Unfortunately, once you've been exposed to this type of herpes virus, it becomes dormant in the body, meaning it does not leave your body so soon. So, in the events wherein your immune system gets compromised, the symptoms of EBV get retriggered or reactivated, causing a whole host of chronic infections and diseases.

However, modern and progressive studies believe that the virus rarely gets reactivated in most healthy individuals—it lies dormant within the body for the rest of your life without any symptoms or complications.

Over the course of the Epstein-Barr Viruses, you may experience four different stages of the virus, and each stage manifests itself with different symptoms and health complications.

In fact, there are more than 60 strains and mutations of these viruses, wherein each strain presents different symptoms as they progress through each stage of virus invasion in your body.

Recent Scientific Advances in Epstein-Barr Virus (EBV) Research

Epstein-Barr Virus (EBV) is a pervasive pathogen that has baffled scientists and clinicians for decades due to its complex and elusive nature. However, recent breakthroughs in research have significantly deepened our understanding of the virus, its role in various diseases, and potential strategies for diagnostic and therapeutic intervention. Below, we explore some of the latest scientific developments in EBV research.

New Diagnostic Tools for Detecting Latent and Reactivated EBV

One of the major challenges in managing EBV has been the difficulty in accurately detecting latent or reactivated infections. Conventional methods, such as serology and polymerase chain reaction (PCR) tests, though effective in diagnosing acute infections, fall short when it comes to identifying dormant EBV within tissues or reactivation events.

Recent advances are changing the diagnostic landscape:

1. **EBV DNA Methylation Assays**

    Researchers are leveraging epigenomic techniques to assess EBV DNA methylation patterns in host cells. Unlike traditional tests that focus solely on the viral load in blood, these assays can detect latent EBV hiding in tissues and cells, providing a more comprehensive understanding of how and where the virus resides in the body.

2. **Next-Generation Sequencing (NGS)**

    NGS allows for the precise tracking of Epstein-Barr genetic material and even identifies specific EBV strains. This technology is being used to understand how different strains impact disease progression and their links to specific conditions, such as cancers and autoimmune diseases.

3. **Biomarker-Based Immunoassays**

    Immunoassays are being refined to detect EBV-specific T-cell responses and early antigen markers that indicate reactivation. These tools offer remarkable sensitivity and specificity, helping clinicians identify early signs of reactivation before severe symptoms emerge.

4. **3D Imaging of Viral Mechanisms**

    Advances in molecular imaging now allow scientists to visualize the interaction between EBV proteins and host cells in three dimensions. This breakthrough provides unprecedented insights into how the virus infiltrates cells and establishes latency, offering new avenues for early detection.

These innovative diagnostic tools are transforming how we detect and manage latent and reactivated EBV infections. By providing deeper insights into the virus's behavior, they pave the way for earlier intervention and improved patient outcomes.

Emerging Therapies for EBV Management

For years, treatment options for EBV were limited to symptomatic relief, with no targeted therapies available. However, ongoing research has uncovered promising therapeutic strategies to combat EBV directly or modulate its effects on the immune system.

1. **Antiviral Drugs Under Development**

    While existing antivirals like acyclovir offer limited success against EBV due to the virus's dormancy mechanisms, new agents are being tested. These drugs aim to disrupt the viral replication cycle even during latent phases. For instance, researchers are exploring inhibitors that target specific EBV proteins, such as the Epstein-Barr nuclear antigen (EBNA) or latent membrane proteins (LMPs).

2. Immune Modulators

Advances in immunology have spurred the development of therapies that enhance the immune system's ability to fight EBV. Immune checkpoint inhibitors, which are commonly used for cancer, are being repurposed to block EBV-infected cells from evading immune surveillance. Similarly, monoclonal antibodies that target viral components are showing promise in clinical trials.

3. Epstein-Barr Vaccines

One of the most exciting developments is the progress toward an EBV vaccine. Researchers are focusing on vaccines that stimulate strong humoral and cellular immune responses against EBV antigens. Phase I clinical trials are demonstrating early safety and efficacy profiles for these vaccine candidates, paving the way for future breakthroughs that could prevent infection altogether.

4. **Gene Therapy and CRISPR Technology**

   Gene-editing tools like CRISPR-Cas9 are being studied for their ability to modify host or viral genes involved in EBV persistence. The goal is to create therapies that can either permanently inactivate EBV in infected cells or enhance the host's antiviral defense mechanisms.

Emerging therapies for EBV management are opening new possibilities, from antiviral drugs and immune modulators to vaccines and gene-editing technologies. These advancements hold the potential to not only treat EBV more effectively but also prevent infections in the future.

Links Between EBV and Chronic Diseases

The role of EBV in triggering or exacerbating chronic and severe illnesses has come under intense scrutiny in recent years. Fresh evidence continues to reveal how this virus is intertwined with conditions that profoundly impact human health.

EBV and Autoimmune Conditions

EBV has long been suspected of contributing to various autoimmune diseases. Recent studies have identified molecular mimicry—the phenomenon where EBV proteins resemble human proteins—as a driving factor behind diseases like multiple sclerosis (MS), lupus, and rheumatoid arthritis.

EBV's ability to disrupt regulatory immune pathways, especially through persistent infection of B-cells, is believed to activate autoimmunity in genetically susceptible individuals.

Links to Cancer

EBV is a known oncogenic virus associated with malignancies such as Hodgkin's lymphoma, Burkitt lymphoma, nasopharyngeal carcinoma, and gastric cancer. The study of EBV-related cancers is providing valuable insights into how the virus reprograms infected cells, leading to unchecked growth and tumor formation. Current research is developing therapies that specifically target EBV-driven tumorigenesis, such as targeted EBV immunotherapies.

EBV and Long COVID

Emerging research has begun to connect EBV reactivation with long COVID. Individuals suffering from prolonged symptoms after recovering from a COVID-19 infection often show markers of EBV reactivation, implicating the virus in fatigue, neurological symptoms, and an overactivated immune system. This association is driving an exploration of antiviral and immunomodulatory treatments to help long COVID patients.

While these scientific advancements are encouraging, translating them into clinical applications remains a complex task. Many of these emerging tools and therapies are still in experimental stages, requiring further validation and large-scale clinical trials. Nevertheless, these findings are setting the stage for a future where EBV infections are easier to detect, manage, and potentially prevent altogether.

By staying at the forefront of research, we inch closer to a world where the Epstein-Barr Virus—long misunderstood—can be effectively tamed, reducing its impact on millions of lives.

The EBV Stages

Now that we have an understanding of the basics behind EBV, let's dive deeper into the different stages of the virus and how it affects the body. In most cases, individuals can experience four different stages of EBV infection:

Stage One of Epstein-Barr

The first stage of Epstein-Barr is called the latent or inactivity phase of EBV infection, wherein the Epstein-Barr viruses infect cells in the body and float in your bloodstream, and remain dormant, doing nothing besides multiplying inside their nuclei awaiting the vulnerable opportunity to launch the real infection.

During this latent or early stage of EBV infection, the disease's cure is not clear because the virus is vulnerable in your body, meaning it's undetectable with no symptoms making it hard for you to fight it off since you won't be aware it exists.

At this stage, the new cases of EBV are sporadic, and the virus typically attacks in a matter of proximity when it detects your stress-related hormones.

For example, the most commonly reported weak moments for the virus to act include:

- When you're physically exhausted for weeks, and you do not give your body a chance to recover
- Your body is deprived of essential nutrients such as Vitamin B12 or Zinc
- If you're undergoing a traumatic emotional event such as the loss or leaving of a loved one
- Another common scenario is when women are experiencing major hormonal changes that occur during pregnancy, childbirth, puberty, or even menopause. Afterward, they may exhibit various symptoms such as fatigue, aches, discomfort, or even depression.

In the context of hormonal changes in women, the Epstein-Barr Virus (EBV) doesn't necessarily exploit weaknesses. Instead, it uses the surge of hormones as a fuel source, turning them into triggers for viral activity.

Put simply, this virus is remarkably patient—almost unnervingly so.

Why? Because EBV can strengthen itself and lie dormant for years, waiting for the right conditions to activate. Factors like the host's immune system play a significant role in determining when this "action period" occurs.

Stage Two of Epstein-Barr

This stage is when the virus exists in your body, which means it is now active and ready to fight your body.

This stage is generally defined by the proliferation of the virus, which may cause your immune system to overreact and generate excessively high amounts of mononucleosis—the famous mono known as "kissing disease" that we grow up hearing about.

That is, in this active stage, mononucleosis typically produces high amounts of formaldehyde, an effect that is often described as radiating.

Therefore, it is a good idea to avoid close contact or exposure to someone else's bodily fluids, from saliva or blood, regardless of their mono status.

And since this stage is the most contagious, your immune system is more likely to experience severe symptoms, and it will try to battle the virus off by sending the cell identifiers to tag and kill the virus cells.

The severity of this battle varies from individual to individual, and it solely depends on the type of EBV strain or variant and the immune system of the "host."

Still, at this stage, mononucleosis can present itself as a mild illness such as tiredness, sore throats, rashes, and headaches for a week or two. As such, you're unlikely to realize what's going on. Thus, you'll blush at the idea of visiting a doctor or having a blood test.

But then again, as the virus gains more access to your body, signs and symptoms can worsen, and you might start having unexplained symptoms all over your body.

The typical symptoms that appear at stage two of Epstein-Barr can include:

- Extremely fatigued
- Intense muscle aches
- Headaches
- Night sweats
- Fever
- Sore throat
- Swollen lymph nodes
- Body rashes
- Swollen liver and enlarged spleen
- Shortness of breath or heavy breathing
- Nausea

If you notice any of these symptoms, don't ignore them because, most likely, it's the onset of the Epstein-Barr virus. Instead, keep a close eye on the signs and call your doctor or take a viral infection test to be sure.

Speaking of the liver and the spleen, during stage two of EBV, the virus progresses rapidly and begins to hide in these major organs. This is because the EBV flourishes in toxins accumulated in these organs. The said toxins are mercury, dioxins, and a wide range of toxins.

Stage Three of Epstein-Barr Virus

The third stage of Epstein-Barr is the most intense now that the virus has slipped into your major organs, including the liver and spleen.

What this means is that, during the third stage, the virus is actively alive in your organs and causing new symptoms. Most likely, it is undetectable since no established tests to detect EBV in the liver, spleen, or major body organs.

The virus is also presently undetected in your bloodstream, making your body assume that it won the battle against the invading viruses present, with the help of white blood cells, and the invader has been destroyed.

At this point, your immune system gets fully restored, but unfortunately, the typical effects of EBV have just begun to get actively aggressive through your body. And because mononucleosis often gets worse and longer than the onset of the virus, this will create more severe problems in the organs, turning the body against you.

Depending on the stage of the EBV variant (typical or aggressive) and how long the virus has been burrowing deep into the liver or spleen, the strain can scar these organs, making them inflamed or enlarged.

And again, it is believed that many doctors fail to connect the dots between the "already passed" EBV infection and its current occupation within your organs.

The burden added to your organs as a result of EBV nesting there can therefore trigger some issues that may include:

- Lupus
- Sluggish liver performance
- Hypothyroidism and an array of thyroid disorders
- Hepatitis C
- Sensitivity to certain foods
- Digestive issues

Without proper management, the burden on these organs can contribute to chronic health conditions, including autoimmune diseases such as lupus.

Stage Four of Epstein-Barr Virus

Typically, the objective goal of the Epstein-Barr virus at this stage is to leave your thyroid gland and cross to your central nervous system and make it inflamed.

This is because the EBV replicated incredibly fast and wore down your thyroid during the third stage. Thankfully, your immune system seems to be alert, hindering this from happening.

However, in the event that you abruptly experience some kind of physical or emotional injury, the virus detects your vulnerability and attempts to exploit your weaknesses causing unexplainable symptoms such as heart palpitations, general body aches, and nerve pains.

The most common injury scenario is an accident, surgery, or physical damage that might leave you feeling unwell for quite some time than expected from the injury.

In fact, this stage is the primary culprit of some mysterious symptoms you might be experiencing, and the worst part of it is the inability of blood tests, X-rays, and MRIs to detect anything wrong, so the symptoms are mistakenly for other illnesses since the doctors aren't aware that the virus is already inflaming the nerves.

Also, when any of your nerves are damaged, it signals the body of its vulnerability and needs repair by triggering the "alarm" hormone that acts as a messenger. And as soon as EBV detects this "disorder hormone," it rushes out quickly to try and attack those damaged nerves.

Remember, when a nerve is injured, its roots pop off out of the nerve sheath, meaning the EBV takes advantage of the openings left, and if it succeeds in grabbing them, it flares up the area and keeps it inflamed for years or even decades.

Some of the symptoms resulting from this stage four viral inflammation can include:

- Muscle pains
- Ongoing fatigue and dizziness
- Blurred vision
- Disturbed sleep
- Night sweats
- Painful tender points
- Insomnia
- Numbness/ tingling in the hands and feet
- Back Pains
- Anxiety
- Asthma
- Heart palpitations

The virus exploits nerve injuries by infiltrating exposed nerve roots, causing persistent inflammation that can last for years or even decades.

How Epstein-Barr Virus (EBV) Affects Your Immune System

The Epstein-Barr Virus (EBV) is more than just the cause behind the common "kissing disease." This tricky virus has a way of hiding in your body and directly interfering with your immune system, which is responsible for protecting you from illnesses. Here's a look at how EBV interacts with the immune system, weakens it over time, and what you can do to strengthen your defenses.

How EBV Impacts T-Cells and B-Cells

Your immune system has different "soldiers" that work to fight off infections. Two of the most important types are T-cells and B-cells. Think of T-cells as the field generals, calling the shots and coordinating the immune response, while B-cells are the factories that produce antibodies to fight off specific threats, like viruses.

When EBV enters your body, it goes straight for your B-cells:

- *Hijacking B-Cells:* EBV infects B-cells, takes over their machinery, and uses them as hiding spots to

evade the immune system. While inside, the virus can multiply quietly or become dormant, waiting for the right moment to reactivate (for example, during periods of stress or illness).
- *Overwhelming T-Cells:* Your T-cells recognize the infected B-cells and try to destroy them. But if there are too many infected cells, your T-cells can become exhausted from fighting, leaving your immune system weaker overall. It's like having too many alarms going off at the same time and not enough people to turn them off.

EBV targets your B-cells, using them to hide and multiply, while overwhelming your T-cells trying to fight back. This weakens your immune system, making it harder to respond to future threats.

Chronic EBV and Weak Immune Defenses

If your body can't fully control the virus, EBV can stick around and cause long-term trouble. Chronic EBV infections can:

- *Keep the Immune System on Overdrive:* Your immune system may stay in a constant state of alert, leading to inflammation and making you feel tired, achy, and unwell over time.
- *Distract the Immune System:* Because your immune system is so busy dealing with EBV, it can become

"distracted" and less effective at keeping other infections or illnesses at bay.
- ***Open the Door to Autoimmune Problems:*** People with chronic EBV may develop autoimmune diseases, where the immune system mistakenly attacks healthy parts of the body. This happens because EBV-infected cells can confuse your immune system into targeting your own tissues.

Chronic EBV can weaken your immune system, leaving you vulnerable to inflammation, infections, and even autoimmune diseases. Understanding its impact is essential for managing symptoms and protecting your overall health.

How to Rebuild and Support Your Immune System

There are plenty of practical ways to help your immune system recover and better handle EBV. Here's how to start:

1. ***Eat Immune-Boosting Foods:*** Focus on nutrient-rich foods that help your body fight off infections. Some great options include:
    - Leafy greens like spinach and kale, which contain vitamins C and E.
    - Citrus fruits, such as oranges and grapefruits, for their immune-boosting vitamin C.
    - Garlic and ginger, which have natural antiviral and anti-inflammatory properties.

2. ***Stay Hydrated:*** Drink plenty of water to help flush out toxins and keep your body functioning well. Herbal teas, like lemon balm or licorice root tea, can also support the immune system while calming inflammation.
3. ***Get Restful Sleep:*** Sleep is essential for repairing your body and recharging your immune system. Aim for 7–9 hours of quality sleep each night, and create a calming bedtime routine to help you wind down.
4. ***Try Gentle Exercise:*** Moderate physical activity can boost circulation and improve immune function. Even simple activities like walking or yoga can do wonders for your overall health.
5. ***Take Immune-Supporting Supplements:*** Certain vitamins and minerals can give your immune system an extra boost. Consider adding:
    - Vitamin C for its infection-fighting power.
    - Zinc to help reduce inflammation and support healing.
    - L-lysine, an amino acid that can suppress viruses like EBV.
6. ***Reduce Stress:*** Stress can weaken your immune defenses and encourage EBV to reactivate. Practice relaxation techniques like deep breathing, mindfulness, or meditation to keep your stress levels in check.
7. ***Consult with Your Doctor:*** If you're dealing with stubborn symptoms, talk to your healthcare provider.

They may recommend antiviral treatments, immune-boosting therapies, or additional strategies to help you recover.

Rebuilding your immune system after dealing with EBV takes time, but with consistent care, you can feel stronger and healthier. A balanced diet, regular rest, and manageable stress levels are key to keeping the virus under control. Remember, your immune system is like a garden—it needs attention, nourishment, and care to thrive. Keep tending to it, and you'll see the results over time.

Health Complications Associated with EBV

The EBV can be transmitted through saliva, making it mistakenly diagnosed as a common cold sore virus. But that's not all it can do. This nasty little bug has been connected with other medical issues, and it is believed to be the common cause of chronic fatigue syndrome (CFS), fibromyalgia, and a slew of other chronic illnesses.

However, the biggest problem with EBV is that it can hide for years before reappearing in the form of illness. By then, you'll have a much bigger fight on your hands than if you'd taken the right action early on.

The most chronic illnesses linked to the aggressive nesting of this virus in your organs are:

- Fibromyalgia
- Chronic Fatigue Syndrome
- Tinnitus
- Rheumatoid Arthritis
- Hepatitis C

- Vertigo and Meniere's Disease
- Multiple Sclerosis
- Neurological complications
- Cancers

EBV is more than just a harmless virus—it's linked to serious chronic illnesses and can remain dormant for years before causing significant health issues. Taking proactive measures early on is key to minimizing its impact on your long-term health.

Mental Health and EBV

Coping with Epstein-Barr Virus (EBV) and its chronic fatigue can impact both your body and mind. This section provides practical tips to boost your mood, improve mental clarity, and enhance your quality of life while managing EBV. You're not alone—there are ways to support your mental well-being alongside your physical health.

Understanding the Psychological Impact of EBV

Living with EBV symptoms can feel isolating and overwhelming. Chronic fatigue may stop you from doing the things you love or spending time with others, leading to feelings of anxiety or depression. On top of that, "brain fog"—things like forgetting details, feeling mentally sluggish, or having trouble focusing—can make everyday tasks harder.

Understanding these effects is the first step. It's important to acknowledge what you're going through without judgment. Be kind to yourself—EBV is a real challenge, but it doesn't define who you are.

Techniques to Manage Anxiety, Depression, and Stress

Here are simple, effective ways to help you better manage the emotional weight of living with EBV.

1. *Use Relaxation Techniques:* Relaxation doesn't just calm your mind—it eases tension in your body too.
    - Deep breathing: Sit quietly and take slow, deep breaths in through your nose and out through your mouth. This can help lower feelings of anxiety.
    - Meditation: Spend 5–10 minutes each day focusing on your breath or listening to calming meditation apps like Calm or Headspace.
    - Gentle yoga or stretching: These activities combine movement and mindfulness, which can reduce both physical and emotional stress.
2. *Practice Gratitude:* It can be hard to focus on the positives when you're not feeling your best, but small acts of gratitude can lift your mood. Try writing down three things you're thankful for each evening, no matter how small—like a sunny day or a supportive friend.

3. ***Talk to Someone:*** It's okay to ask for help. Whether it's a trusted friend, a family member, or a counselor, sharing what you're going through can lighten the emotional load. Sometimes, just being heard is enough to feel better.

Managing anxiety, depression, and stress takes small, consistent steps like practicing relaxation, gratitude, and reaching out for support. By incorporating these techniques into your routine, you can create a more balanced and positive mindset over time.

Tips for Combating "Brain Fog"

"Brain fog," or mental cloudiness, is a common but frustrating symptom of EBV. Here are some helpful strategies to stay sharp and focused.

1. ***Snack Smart:*** Choose snacks that fuel your brain, like nuts, seeds, fresh fruits, or dark leafy greens. These foods provide the nutrients your brain needs to function better.
2. ***Stay Hydrated:*** Surprisingly, dehydration can make brain fog worse. Drink plenty of water throughout the day, and limit caffeine or sugary drinks that might leave you feeling even more sluggish later on.
3. ***Break Big Tasks Into Smaller Steps:*** If focusing feels impossible, don't force it. Instead, break big tasks into bite-sized pieces and tackle them one at a time.

Celebrate progress, no matter how small—it's all movement in the right direction.
4. ***Take Brain Breaks:*** When your attention starts to slip, don't push through it. Stand up, take a quick walk, or close your eyes for a few minutes. Short breaks often restore focus and help you feel clearer.

By making small, intentional changes like eating brain-friendly snacks, staying hydrated, and taking breaks, you can manage brain fog more effectively. Remember, progress takes time—be kind to yourself as you work toward feeling sharper and more focused.

EBV and Sleep Disturbances

EBV can seriously mess with your sleep—whether it's trouble falling asleep, staying asleep, or feeling unrefreshed even after sleeping. Lack of rest doesn't just leave you tired—it can also worsen anxiety, depression, and brain fog.

How to Improve Sleep Quality

- ***Create a Routine:*** Go to bed and wake up at the same time every day, even on weekends. This helps regulate your body's internal clock.
- ***Limit Screen Time:*** Avoid screens (like your phone or TV) for at least an hour before bedtime. The blue light can interfere with natural sleep hormones.

- ***Try Relaxing Activities:*** Read a calming book, take a warm bath, or listen to soothing music before bed to help signal to your brain that it's time to wind down.
- ***Keep the Bedroom Calm:*** Make your bedroom dark, quiet, and cool. If noise is an issue, try white noise machines or earplugs.
- ***Experiment With Natural Sleep Aids:*** Herbal teas like chamomile or supplements like magnesium may improve sleep. Always consult a healthcare provider before trying new supplements.

Living with EBV can affect mental health, but small steps like deep breathing, healthy snacks, and better sleep can help. Healing takes time—be kind to yourself, lean on loved ones, and focus on moments of joy to feel stronger each day.

Practical Stress Management Programs for EBV Recovery

Managing stress is crucial for breaking the cycle of Epstein-Barr Virus (EBV) reactivations and supporting recovery. This chapter provides practical techniques like mindfulness challenges and breathing exercises to help reduce stress, improve mental well-being, and promote healing.

How Chronic Stress Triggers EBV Reactivation

Chronic stress weakens the immune system, allowing dormant EBV to reactivate and cause symptoms like fatigue and brain fog. Managing stress both mentally and physically can help break this cycle and prevent EBV flare-ups.

A 30-Day Mindfulness Challenge for EBV Recovery

Mindfulness is a proven way to reduce stress, calm your nervous system, and improve mental clarity. Over the next 30 days, commit to small daily practices to bring more focus and calm into your life.

Week 1 - Starting Small

- Day 1–7 Focus: Commit to 5 minutes of mindfulness a day.
- Every morning, sit in a quiet space and focus on your breathing. Inhale for 4 counts, hold for 4 counts, and exhale for 6 counts.
- At the end of each session, take a moment to notice how your body feels.

Week 2 - Gratitude and Awareness

- Day 8–14 Focus: Add gratitude to your mindfulness practice.
- Each evening, write down three things you're grateful for. These can be as simple as enjoying a quiet moment or having a supportive friend.
- Reflect on this list during your mindfulness sessions to cultivate a positive mindset.

Week 3 - Mindful Movement

- Day 15–21 Focus: Incorporate gentle movement into your mindfulness practice.
- Try yoga or stretching exercises that align with your breathing. Poses like Child's Pose or seated forward

folds help release muscle tension associated with stress.

Week 4 - Building Consistency
- Day 22–30 Focus: Extend mindfulness into daily life.
- Practice mindful eating by savoring each bite at meals. Limit distractions like phones or TV.
- Pause for 1–2 minutes of deep breathing before stressful tasks or conversations.

By the end of 30 days, these small habit changes will become part of your routine, helping you maintain a calmer, more focused state even in challenging moments.

Daily Breathing Exercises to Support Your Nervous System

Deep breathing can work wonders for calming your nervous system. Try these exercises daily or during moments of stress to feel more grounded and relaxed.

1. **Diaphragmatic Breathing (Belly Breathing)**
    - Sit in a comfortable position and place one hand on your stomach.
    - Breathe in deeply through your nose, feeling your stomach rise under your hand.
    - Exhale slowly through pursed lips, allowing your stomach to fall.

- Repeat for 5 minutes to lower cortisol levels and relax your body.

2. **Box Breathing**
   - Breathe in through your nose for 4 counts.
   - Hold your breath for 4 counts.
   - Exhale through your mouth for 4 counts.
   - Hold your breath again for 4 counts.
   - Repeat this cycle for 3–5 minutes. Box breathing promotes a sense of control and eases anxious thoughts.

3. **Alternate Nostril Breathing**
   - Use your thumb to close your right nostril.
   - Breathe in through your left nostril, then close it with your ring finger. Release your thumb to exhale through your right nostril.
   - Switch sides and repeat for 5–10 cycles.
   - This technique balances your nervous system, helping you feel both energized and calm.

These simple exercises can be practiced any time—first thing in the morning, before bed, or whenever you need a quick reset.

Breaking the Cycle of Stress and EBV Reactivation

The link between chronic stress and EBV makes it essential to address stress at its root. Here are practical steps to help break the cycle and support your recovery.

1. ***Rest and Prioritize Sleep:*** Good sleep is essential for recovery. Poor rest increases stress and weakens the immune system. Stick to a consistent schedule, create a calming bedtime routine, and avoid screens before bed.
2. ***Set Boundaries:*** Learn to say "no" to over-commitment. Reduce stress by cutting back on draining obligations. Focus on activities you enjoy, like spending time in nature, journaling, or simply resting.
3. ***Nourish Your Body:*** Stress depletes essential nutrients. Support yourself with a nutrient-rich diet full of fresh fruits, veggies, healthy fats, and anti-inflammatory herbs like lemon balm and ginger.
4. ***Seek Social Support:*** Isolation can add to stress. Reach out to a friend, family member, or support group. Sharing your experiences with someone who understands can ease the emotional burden of managing EBV.

Managing stress with EBV can feel challenging, but small, consistent efforts like mindfulness and calming breathing techniques can help break the stress-reactivation cycle. Be patient, trust the process, and celebrate progress as you work toward healing and peace of mind.

Natural Epstein-Barr Treatment Protocols

Since there is no modern treatment to suppress EBV, some practitioners and naturopaths agree that you can incorporate natural protocols in your lifestyle to help suppress the virus while creating an environment where the EBV antibodies are unlikely to thrive.

But before we get to the rundown of these protocols, let's first understand how to diagnose this little bug.

Transmission and Diagnosis

According to the Centers for Disease Control and Prevention (CDC), EBV can be transmitted through saliva. The most common routes of infection include kissing, coughing (and sneezing) on someone, and sharing items such as cigarettes, lip balm, or glasses that can transmit the virus.

The virus can also be transmitted from pregnant women to their unborn children if the mother has the virus.

However, in some cases, the virus can be spread through organ transplantation procedures, bodily fluids such as semen during sexual contact, and through children's toys that have been drooled on.

Diagnosing the potential presence of Epstein-Barr Virus in the body is not always easy since the symptoms are mistakenly linked to other illnesses.

However, the presence of antibodies believed to cause EBV can be confirmed through a blood test, with the common one known as the monospot test.

In addition to this type of test, your doctor will request more specific antibodies blood tests, including the following:

- *Viral Capsid antigen.* The VCA antibodies appear during the latent stages of the infection, with anti-VCA IgM disappearing in a few weeks while the anti-VCA IgG becomes persistent for life.
- *Early antigen or EA.* Typically, the EA antibodies will surface during the active phase of the infection. And even though these antibodies may remain in your body for several months, they are undetectable. Some people can be persistent even for years.

- ***EBV nuclear antigen or (EBNA).*** The antibodies of this type slowly surface a few months after the infection invasion in the body and can be easily detected.

In addition to these blood tests, the practitioner will consider other factors such as your overall health or the presence of any other underlying medical condition to make a diagnosis.

Natural Treatment for EBV Infections

As I had earlier stated, there is no prescribed treatment or vaccine for EBV infection, but still, there are other natural EBV treatment steps to help you regain your health and energy back over time.

With that being said, this four-part program can help replenish your immune system, making it perform its tasks of keeping the virus at bay effectively.

Step 1: Drinking Plenty of Fluids

If you want to know how to treat the Epstein-Barr virus naturally, one of the most important steps is to stay hydrated. Our bodies are made up of 60% water, and we need a constant supply of it to function properly.

Drinking plenty of water helps flush out harmful waste and toxins from your body, which is vital for getting rid of viruses like the Epstein-Barr virus.

Besides, water regulates our body temperature, transports nutrients to the cells, helps digestion, and helps collagen production. So, if you're feeling sick, you should drink plenty of water and other fluids such as fruit and vegetable juices to help prevent dehydration.

Step 2: Get Quality Restorative Rest

One of the strangest things about EBV is that you constantly feel weary and tired, yet you cannot sleep—a natural tendency similar to that of a night owl.

And unfortunately, lack of adequate sleep or rest suppresses your immune system and triggers hormonal changes in your body, resulting in EBV reactivation.

So, whenever you feel tired, constantly try to incorporate a relaxation technique in your nighttime routine and diligently stick to it to reset your already stressed immune system.

Along with that, be gentle to yourself and get a little more restorative sleep whenever you feel you need it. This will help your body to recover and repair itself naturally.

Step 3: Detoxify Your Body to Support The Immune System

Detoxing can help manage Epstein-Barr Virus (EBV) by supporting the liver and kidneys, reducing toxins, and easing inflammation. This step covers detox strategies, including 7-

or 14-day plans, foods, teas, supplements, and protocols for heavy metal removal to alleviate EBV symptoms.

How Detoxification Supports EBV Recovery

Detoxification happens in two main phases within the liver and kidneys.

- *Phase I:* The liver processes toxins and converts them into substances that can be eliminated.
- *Phase II:* These neutralized toxins are excreted through the kidneys or intestines.

If these detox processes are slowed (due to toxins or inflammation), your body struggles to flush out waste, allowing EBV to thrive. Detoxification helps clear harmful substances like heavy metals and inflammatory antibodies linked to EBV, paving the way for your immune system to recover and function optimally.

7- or 14-Day Detox Plan for EBV Support

Follow this structured plan to safely and effectively detoxify your body, helping ease symptoms of EBV like fatigue and inflammation.

Day 1–7 (Preparation and Kidney/Liver Support)

Morning Routine

- Start each day with 16–20 oz of warm lemon water to stimulate your liver's detox pathways and aid digestion.
- Drink fresh celery juice (16 oz) immediately after, as it's packed with mineral salts that support liver and kidney health while fighting EBV.

Meals

- Focus on anti-inflammatory and alkaline foods such as leafy greens (spinach, kale), cruciferous vegetables (broccoli, cauliflower), and hydrating fruits like cucumbers and watermelon. These foods help neutralize acidity and promote organ function.
- Add wild blueberries to smoothies or snacks—these berries help cleanse the liver and brain of EBV neurotoxins.
- Incorporate healthy fats like avocado, flaxseeds, or chia seeds for hormone balance and inflammation reduction.

Teas and Drinks

- Sip dandelion root tea to support your liver and kidneys.
- Use burdock root tea for additional gentle detoxification and inflammation relief.

Supplements

- Milk Thistle: Aids liver repair and supports Phase I and II detoxification.
- Nettle Leaf: Promotes kidney function and cleanses the blood.
- Vitamin C: Flushes toxins while improving immune defenses against EBV.

Self-Care

End each day with a warm detox bath containing Epsom salt (2 cups) or bentonite clay (1/2 cup). These baths draw toxins out of the skin while relaxing sore muscles.

Day 8–14 (Focus on Heavy Metal Detox)

Morning Routine

Continue with warm lemon water and celery juice but add 1–2 teaspoons of cilantro juice or chopped fresh cilantro to your smoothies. Cilantro is an effective natural chelating agent for heavy metals.

Meals

- Feature ingredients that bind heavy metals, such as spirulina and wild blueberries, in your meals or shakes. These superfoods capture and help eliminate toxins. Include them in nutrient-packed smoothies with a handful of spinach and a banana for sweetness.

- Incorporate Omega-3-rich foods like walnuts and wild-caught salmon, which reduce inflammation further.

Teas and Drinks

- Increase detoxification with red clover tea, known to cleanse the blood and support skin detox.
- Lemon balm tea can soothe nerves while also reducing viral activity.

Supplements

- **Chlorella:** A powerful detoxifier that works alongside spirulina to remove heavy metals from your system.
- **Selenium:** Boosts liver health and prevents oxidative stress caused by heavy metals.
- **L-Glutathione:** Supports liver enzymes and acts as a master antioxidant to protect against toxins.

Self-Care

Continue detox baths and add dry brushing before bathing to stimulate your lymphatic system, helping with additional toxin elimination.

EBV-Detox Superfoods and Teas

Below are some highly beneficial ingredients to incorporate during your detox.

Liver and Kidney Cleansing Foods

- **Beets:** Rich in betaine, which aids liver detoxification and regenerates healthy liver cells.
- **Parsley:** A natural kidney cleanser and heavy-metal chelator—add it to juices, soups, or salads.
- **Cranberries:** Improve urinary tract health and help eliminate toxins from the kidneys.

Healing Herbal Teas

- **Ginger Tea:** Boosts circulation and promotes toxin removal through perspiration and the digestive tract.
- **Chamomile Tea:** Reduces inflammation and supports better sleep during the detox phase.

Heavy Metal Detox Protocols

Heavy metals like mercury and aluminum can feed EBV and worsen symptoms. Removing these toxins is critical for recovery.

Key Heavy Metal Cleansers:

- Cilantro & Spirulina: Both capture metals stored in your organs and carry them out of the body. Use them together for the best results.
- Algae-Based Detox: Chlorella simultaneously binds to heavy metals and supplies chlorophyll to aid liver repair.
- Apple Pectin: Found in apples, it helps remove metals from the bloodstream and supports better digestion.

How to Add Them

- Blend cilantro, spirulina, and wild blueberries into a morning smoothie for a concentrated detox drink.
- Enjoy a spirulina latte with almond milk and a touch of honey for something warm and soothing.

Final Tips for a Successful EBV Detox

- *Stay Hydrated:* Water is essential for flushing toxins through your kidneys—drink at least 8 glasses per day.
- *Avoid Toxins in Your Environment:* Cut back on exposure to household chemicals, heavily processed foods, alcohol, and cigarette smoke.
- *Listen to Your Body:* If you feel overly fatigued from detoxing, slow down. Give your body time to adjust.

By following this easy-to-implement detox plan, flooding your diet with healing foods, and taking key supplements, you'll create a stronger foundation for both detoxification and immune support as your body fights EBV. Small efforts each day add up, setting you on the path to recovery. Every step you take gets you closer to feeling better.

Step 4: Moderate Exercises

Staying active is crucial when fighting EBV, as movement boosts circulation and supports your immune system. Moderate exercise, like a 15-minute walk or 30 minutes of activity daily, helps your body combat this energy-draining virus by keeping blood flow, muscles, and lymph in motion.

Moderate exercises can also play a role in regulating your body's response to stress. For example, the endorphins released during exercise can reduce your body's production of the stress hormone cortisol. This boosts your body's stress response, which can ultimately help restore and reset your immune system.

However, given the overall benefits of this four-part program, other patients with EBV have been confirmed to combine the Epstein-Barr diet with herbs and supplements to treat the recurrent or chronic virus.

Incorporating Herbal Remedies into Daily Life for EBV Management

Managing Epstein-Barr Virus (EBV) can be supported with herbs and natural supplements, which offer antiviral, immune-boosting, and anti-inflammatory benefits. This chapter provides practical tips on using herbal remedies, including infusions, tinctures, and teas, alongside DIY recipes and safety advice to enhance your healing process.

The Power of Herbs in EBV Management

Certain herbs are stars when it comes to combating EBV. They're filled with compounds that strengthen the immune system, calm inflammation, and even target EBV cells directly. Here are three key herbs you can easily add to your routine and their benefits:

- ***Lemon Balm:*** Known for its antiviral and calming properties, lemon balm can reduce stress on the nervous system while directly fighting the EBV virus.

- *Licorice Root:* This herb has potent antiviral and anti-inflammatory effects, supporting adrenal health while managing EBV-related fatigue.
- *Astragalus:* Astragalus strengthens the immune system, combats viral replication, and helps with energy restoration.

How to Incorporate Herbs Into Daily Life

Herbs are versatile and can be prepared in a variety of ways to suit your taste and lifestyle. Below are three key methods you can try.

1. *Herbal Infusions:* An infusion is a strong water-based preparation that extracts compounds from dried herbs. It's ideal for tough leaves, flowers, or stems.

   How to Prepare:
   - Add 1–2 tablespoons of dried herbs (e.g., lemon balm or astragalus) to a heat-safe jar or teapot.
   - Pour 2 cups of boiling water over the herbs.
   - Cover and steep for 20–30 minutes for maximum potency.
   - Strain the liquid and drink warm or store in the fridge for later use (up to 48 hours).

   Herbal infusions are perfect for sipping throughout the day, especially when you need a calm boost or antiviral support.

2. ***Herbal Tinctures:*** Tinctures are highly concentrated herbal extracts made with alcohol or glycerin. They're convenient if you're on the go or prefer a quick method.

   How to Prepare:

   - Fill a clean jar with fresh or dried herbs. (For example, use licorice root or astragalus root.)
   - Pour vodka (or glycerin for an alcohol-free version) over the herbs, covering them completely.
   - Seal the jar and store it in a cool, dark place for 4–6 weeks, shaking it gently every day.
   - Strain the mixture through cheesecloth or a fine sieve. Keep the liquid in a labeled glass dropper bottle.

   How to Use: Add 1–2 droppers of tincture to water or tea 2–3 times a day.

3. ***Herbal Teas:*** Teas offer a quick and easy way to enjoy the benefits of EBV-supportive herbs.

   How to Prepare:

   - Use 1 teaspoon of dried herbs or 1 tablespoon of fresh herbs per cup of water.
   - Steep in hot water for 5–10 minutes, depending on the herb and your taste preference.

- Sweeten with honey if desired.

Teas are best for milder herbs like lemon balm, offering both antiviral support and relaxation when consumed daily.

DIY Recipes for EBV-Supportive Herbs

Here are some simple recipes to try at home using lemon balm, licorice root, and astragalus.

Lemon Balm Calming Tea

Ingredients:

- 1 teaspoon dried lemon balm
- 1 cup hot water
- 1 teaspoon honey (optional)

Instructions:

1. Add lemon balm to a cup and pour hot water over it.
2. Steep for 10 minutes.
3. Strain, optionally sweeten, and enjoy before bed or anytime you feel stressed.

Licorice Root Immune Boost Tincture

Ingredients:

- Dried licorice root
- Vodka (at least 40% alcohol)

Instructions:

1. Fill a glass jar one-third full with licorice root.
2. Pour vodka over the root, covering it by at least an inch.
3. Seal and store for 4–6 weeks, shaking daily.
4. Strain and keep in a tincture bottle. Take 1–2 droppers daily in water.

Astragalus and Ginger Energy Booster Infusion

Ingredients:

- 2 tablespoons dried astragalus root
- 1-inch piece of fresh ginger, sliced
- 4 cups water

Instructions:

1. Add astragalus and ginger to a pot of water.
2. Simmer on low heat for 20 minutes.
3. Strain and drink warm throughout the day.

Dosage and Safety Precautions

While herbs are natural, they can still be potent and should be used mindfully.

1. *Start Small:* If you're new to an herb, start with small amounts to ensure you don't have any sensitivities.
2. *Stick to Recommended Dosages:*
    - Lemon Balm Tea: 1–3 cups daily.
    - Astragalus Infusion/Tincture: No more than 10 grams of dried herb daily or according to tincture dosing guidelines.
    - Licorice Root Tincture/Tea: Limit use to a few weeks to avoid side effects like elevated blood pressure.

3. ***Consult Your Doctor:*** Especially if you're pregnant, breastfeeding, or taking medications. Some herbs can interfere with certain conditions or treatments.
4. ***Take Breaks:*** For long-term use, cycle herbs with breaks (e.g., use for 3 weeks, pause for 1 week).

Herbal remedies like lemon balm, licorice root, and astragalus can support EBV management by boosting immunity, reducing inflammation, and promoting balance. Start small and listen to your body as these natural additions help enhance your healing journey.

Comprehensive Guide to Supplements for EBV Recovery

Epstein-Barr Virus (EBV) can lead to fatigue, stress, and immune issues, but supplements like selenium, L-lysine, zinc, and adaptogens such as ashwagandha and holy basil can support recovery. This chapter highlights the best supplements, along with dosage tips and precautions for safe and effective use.

Key Supplements for EBV Recovery

1. *Selenium:* Selenium is a powerful mineral that helps your body fight viruses—like EBV—while protecting your nervous system from damage. It's also an antioxidant, meaning it reduces inflammation caused by EBV.
    - **Optimal Dosage:** 100–200 mcg (micrograms) per day.
    - **How It Helps:** Selenium strengthens your immune system and keeps oxidative stress in check, helping your body recover faster.

- **Tip:** Brazil nuts are a great natural source of selenium. One or two nuts a day can meet your daily needs if you prefer a food-based approach.
2. *L-Lysine:* L-lysine is an essential amino acid, which means your body can't make it on its own—you have to get it from food or supplements. It works by lowering viral activity and reducing inflammation that EBV often causes.
    - **Optimal Dosage:** 1,000–3,000 mg (milligrams) per day. Higher doses may be recommended during EBV flare-ups, but speak to your doctor first.
    - **How It Helps:** This supplement not only fights the virus but also soothes inflammation in your central nervous system, minimizing symptoms like fatigue and brain fog.
    - **Tip:** Pair L-lysine supplements with a healthy diet that's low in arginine-rich foods (like nuts and seeds), as too much arginine can feed the virus.
3. *Zinc:* Zinc is essential for immune health, and it plays a unique role in protecting your thyroid from the harmful by-products of EBV. It's also known for shortening the duration of illnesses and speeding up recovery.

- **Optimal Dosage:** 15–30 mg per day. For flare-ups, your doctor may recommend up to 50 mg a day for a short period.
- **How It Helps:** Zinc boosts your immunity, repairs damaged tissues, and reduces the virus's impact on your thyroid.
- **Tip:** Zinc is best absorbed on an empty stomach but can cause nausea in some people. If this happens, take it with food.

Incorporating key supplements like selenium, L-lysine, and zinc can significantly support your recovery from EBV by boosting immunity, reducing inflammation, and protecting your nervous system. Always consult with your doctor to determine the right dosage and ensure these supplements fit your specific needs.

The Role of Adaptogens in EBV Recovery

Adaptogens are a group of herbs that help your body handle stress while boosting your immune system. Since stress is a common trigger for EBV flare-ups, adaptogens like ashwagandha and holy basil can be incredibly helpful.

1. *Ashwagandha:* Ashwagandha is often called the "stress herb" because it calms the nervous system and reduces anxiety. It also supports healthy adrenal function, making it excellent for tackling EBV-induced fatigue.

- **Optimal Dosage:** 300–600 mg per day. Look for standardized extracts to ensure potency.
- **How It Helps:** Ashwagandha balances cortisol levels (your stress hormone) and keeps inflammation at bay, helping your body recover more effectively.
- **Tip:** Take ashwagandha before bed for better sleep, as it promotes relaxation.

2. *Holy Basil (Tulsi):* Holy basil is another adaptogen known for its calming and antiviral properties. It helps your body fight the virus while reducing chronic stress.
   - **Optimal Dosage:** 400–500 mg per day, or drink 1–2 cups of holy basil tea daily.
   - **How It Helps:** Holy basil reduces inflammation and supports your immune response, while also easing mental stress caused by EBV symptoms.
   - **Tip:** Tulsi tea is a gentle and soothing way to include this adaptogen in your day.

Adaptogens like ashwagandha and holy basil can play a key role in managing stress and boosting your immune system during EBV recovery. By reducing inflammation and supporting adrenal health, they help your body heal more effectively while easing fatigue and mental stress.

Precautions for Combining Supplements with Medications

While supplements can be incredibly helpful, it's important to use them safely—especially if you're taking medications or managing other health conditions.

1. *Talk to Your Doctor First:* Always consult with your healthcare provider before starting any new supplements, especially if you're on medications like blood thinners, thyroid medication, or antidepressants.
2. *Avoid Overlapping Ingredients:* Many multivitamins contain zinc, selenium, or other nutrients discussed here. Check the labels to avoid taking too much of any one nutrient.
3. *Take Breaks with Adaptogens:* Adaptogens are safe for most people, but they work best when cycled. For example, use them for 3–4 weeks, then take a one-week break to prevent your body from building a tolerance.
4. *Be Aware of Interactions*
   - **Zinc and Antibiotics:** Zinc can reduce the absorption of certain antibiotics, so space out these medications by a few hours.
   - **Ashwagandha and Sedatives:** Ashwagandha may enhance the effects of sedatives, so avoid taking them together without medical advice.

Supplements and adaptogens can support EBV recovery by reducing inflammation, managing stress, and boosting your body's defenses. Introduce them one at a time, stay consistent, and pair them with good nutrition and stress management for gradual healing.

Customized Nutrition Plans for Different EBV Stages

Epstein-Barr Virus (EBV) is a complex virus that can impact various systems in the body depending on its stage. Whether it's lingering quietly in a latent state or actively causing symptoms, what you eat can significantly influence how your body copes and heals. By tailoring your nutrition plan to the specific EBV stage, you can support your immune system, reduce inflammation, and improve overall well-being.

Here's a guide to understanding the stages of EBV—latent, active, organ-involved, and nervous system—and how to adjust your diet for each one.

Stage 1: Latent Stage

The latent stage of EBV is when the virus is dormant in your body. While it's not actively causing symptoms, the immune system should stay vigilant. A diet that promotes overall wellness, reduces oxidative stress, and keeps inflammation low is ideal.

Foods to Eat

- *Antioxidant-rich produce:* Blueberries, spinach, kale, and sweet potatoes are packed with micronutrients that keep the immune system strong.
- *Healthy fats:* Avocados, olive oil, and nuts help reduce systemic inflammation and support cellular repair.
- *Gut-friendly foods:* Fermented options like yogurt, kefir, and kimchi aid digestion, crucial for immune health.

Foods to Avoid

- *High-sugar foods:* Processed sweets can suppress your immune system and feed harmful gut bacteria.
- *Refined carbs:* White bread, sugary cereals, and pastries can trigger inflammation.
- *Processed meats:* Deli meats and sausages may promote inflammation due to their preservatives.

Sample Meal Plan for Latent Stage

Breakfast: Greek yogurt topped with blueberries, walnuts, and a drizzle of honey.

Lunch: Grilled chicken salad with mixed greens, avocado, cherry tomatoes, cucumber, olive oil, and lemon dressing.

Snack: Carrot sticks with hummus.

Dinner: Baked salmon with a side of roasted sweet potatoes and steamed broccoli.

Bedtime Drink: Chamomile tea for relaxation.

Stage 2: Active Stage

During an active EBV infection, you're likely battling fatigue, fever, and overall malaise. The focus here is on anti-inflammatory and immune-supportive foods to help the body recover more quickly.

Foods to Eat

- ***Immune-boosting herbs:*** Garlic, ginger, and turmeric can combat inflammation and support healing.
- ***Protein sources:*** Lean proteins like turkey, eggs, tofu, or legumes are essential for recovery.
- ***Vitamin C-rich fruits:*** Oranges, kiwis, and strawberries can boost your immune system.

Foods to Avoid

- ***High-fat fried foods:*** These can suppress immune function and trigger gut imbalances.
- ***Dairy (for some people):*** It may increase mucus production, which could worsen symptoms.
- ***Alcohol:*** It weakens the immune system and prolongs the recovery process.

Sample Meal Plan for Active Stage

Breakfast: Warm oatmeal cooked with almond milk, topped with banana slices, chia seeds, and a sprinkle of cinnamon.

Lunch: Lentil soup with spinach and a side of whole-grain toast.

Snack: A handful of mixed nuts and a small orange.

Dinner: Grilled turkey breast served with brown rice, sautéed zucchini, and garlic.

Bedtime Drink: Warm ginger and turmeric tea with a squeeze of lemon.

Stage 3: Organ-Involved Stage

When EBV affects organs—like the liver or spleen—your diet should support detoxification and reduce strain on these vital systems. You'll want nutrient-dense, easy-to-digest meals to aid the body's repair process.

Foods to Eat

- *Liver-supportive foods:* Beets, leafy greens, and artichokes help detoxify and support the liver.
- *Plant-based proteins:* Lentils, chickpeas, and hemp seeds are easier on the system than heavy animal proteins.
- *Hydrating liquids:* Coconut water, herbal teas, and bone broth keep you hydrated and aid detoxification.

Foods to Avoid

- *High-fat meats:* Red meat and fried foods can overburden the liver.

- *Caffeine:* Too much can be hard on the liver and spleen while dehydrating you.
- *Processed oils:* Refined vegetable oils can promote inflammation.

Sample Meal Plan for Organ-Involved Stage

Breakfast: Green smoothie with spinach, cucumber, celery, apple, and lemon juice.

Lunch: Quinoa salad with roasted beets, arugula, walnuts, and a tahini-lemon dressing.

Snack: Apple slices with almond butter.

Dinner: Steamed cod with a side of mashed cauliflower and lightly sautéed asparagus.

Bedtime Drink: Peppermint tea to soothe digestion.

Stage 4: Nervous System Stage

When EBV impacts the nervous system, symptoms like brain fog, anxiety, or nervous system inflammation are common. The diet here should focus on foods that calm the nervous system and provide steady energy.

Foods to Eat

- *Omega-3s:* Fatty fish like salmon or flax seeds nourish the brain and reduce nerve-related inflammation.

- *Magnesium-rich foods:* Dark chocolate, almonds, and spinach help relax the nervous system.
- *Low-GI carbs:* Sweet potatoes and quinoa keep blood sugar stable, which is crucial for brain health.

Foods to Avoid

- *Artificial additives:* Certain preservatives and colorings can exacerbate neuroinflammation.
- *High-sugar snacks:* Blood sugar swings can worsen brain fog and fatigue.
- *Trans fats:* These can impair cognitive function and nerve signaling.

Sample Meal Plan for Nervous System Stage

Breakfast: Scrambled eggs with spinach and a side of sweet potato hash.

Lunch: Grilled mackerel with a quinoa and kale salad drizzled with olive oil.

Snack: A piece of dark chocolate and a handful of almonds.

Dinner: Roasted chicken with wild rice and a medley of sautéed bell peppers and zucchini.

Bedtime Drink: Warm almond milk with a pinch of cinnamon and nutmeg.

Managing EBV symptoms can feel overwhelming, but the right nutrition plan for each stage can help your body heal and feel stronger. Simple dietary changes, focused on nourishing and anti-inflammatory foods, go a long way in supporting your immune system and reducing the impact of this virus on your life. Listen to your body, adjust based on how you feel, and remember that even small shifts in your diet can make a big difference.

The Epstein-Barr Diet: Supporting Your Body with Nutrition

Managing Epstein-Barr Virus (EBV) goes beyond medical treatments—nutrition plays a key role. A nutrient-rich diet can help reduce symptoms, restore energy, and strengthen the immune system. This guide covers healing foods, helpful herbs and supplements, and what to avoid to support recovery.

How Diet Helps with EBV

- Boosts your immune system to fight EBV directly.
- Reduces EBV neurotoxins that harm your liver, brain, and nervous system.
- Restores nutrients and balances pH levels to help your body heal.

Below, we explore the best foods to eat, the supplements to include, and the foods to avoid when building your EBV diet plan.

EBV Healing Foods

Certain foods are rich in nutrients that can directly or indirectly help your body fight EBV. These foods heal, detoxify, and strengthen different systems in your body, reducing the virus's impact over time.

1. **Wild Blueberries**

   Wild blueberries are among the most powerful foods for healing. Packed with anthocyanins, these tiny fruits are potent antioxidants that reduce inflammation and repair your central nervous system. Wild blueberries can also help flush EBV neurotoxins out of the liver and brain. Add them to smoothies, oatmeal, or eat them as a snack to reap their benefits.

2. **Celery**

   Celery is not just hydrating—it's also rich in sodium cluster salts that inhibit EBV growth in the body. It boosts hydrochloric acid in your gut, improving digestion and nutrient absorption. Drinking fresh celery juice daily is a great way to support your immune system and replenish mineral salts in the central nervous system.

3. **Asparagus**

   Asparagus is a powerhouse of antioxidants and alkalizing agents. It reduces the replication of EBV in the liver and spleen and helps balance the body's pH levels to lower viral activity. Enjoy it steamed, roasted, or added to soups and salads.

4. **Spinach and Kale**

   Leafy greens like spinach and kale are extraordinarily alkalizing and provide essential micronutrients to the nervous system. Kale, in particular, is loaded with alkaloids that protect and strengthen your immune system against EBV.

5. **Parsley**

   Parsley is a natural detoxifier and heavy-metal chelator. It clears out toxic metals like copper and aluminum, which feed EBV and trigger inflammation. Parsley also enhances bile flow in the liver, helping it detox effectively.

6. **Garlic and Ginger**

   Both garlic and ginger are antiviral, anti-inflammatory, and antibacterial. Garlic specifically combats EBV co-factors like streptococcus, which can lead to secondary infections. Ginger supports nutrient assimilation and reduces inflammation-related discomfort.

7. **Sprouts**

   Sprouts are bursting with zinc and selenium, two critical nutrients for immune health. These elevated biotics can prevent EBV from gaining ground in the body while enhancing your system's natural defenses. Add them to salads, sandwiches, or grain bowls.

8. **Lettuce**

   Lettuce is an often-overlooked gem with magnesium and alkaline minerals that rebalance your body's pH. It also promotes digestive health and supports detoxification of EBV from the liver.

Incorporating these healing foods into your diet can help detoxify, strengthen your body, and reduce EBV's impact over time. Small, consistent changes can make a big difference in supporting your immune system and overall health.

Foods to Avoid

Certain foods feed EBV or exacerbate its symptoms. Avoiding these can prevent flare-ups and give your body the best chance to heal.

1. *Yeast-Based Foods:* Yeast-based foods can feed harmful bacteria and promote an imbalanced gut environment, which helps EBV flourish.
2. *Processed Foods:* Highly processed snacks, ready meals, and fast food are full of preservatives and

chemicals that burden the liver and promote inflammation.
3. ***Refined Sugars:*** Sugar feeds EBV directly while suppressing your immune system. Steer clear of candies, baked goods, and sugary drinks.
4. ***Red Meat:*** Red meat creates an acidic environment in your body and overburdens the liver, which is trying to detox. Stick to lean proteins or plant-based alternatives.
5. ***Beans and Legumes:*** Beans, while usually nutritious, can create excess gas and digestive strain during EBV healing phases. If your symptoms are manageable, reintroduce them gradually.
6. ***Coffee and Alcohol:*** Both coffee and alcohol stress the liver and dehydrate the body, making healing more difficult. Opt for herbal teas or hydrating beverages like coconut water instead.
7. ***High-Sodium and Spicy Foods:*** Salty and spicy foods can irritate your stomach lining and worsen inflammation, making it harder for your body to heal.

Recovering from Epstein-Barr Virus takes time, but a nutrient-dense, anti-inflammatory diet can support healing. Focus on wholesome foods, helpful supplements, and avoiding triggers. Simple changes, like starting your day with celery juice or choosing unprocessed meals, can make a big impact. Be patient, listen to your body, and trust the process for long-term health.

Epstein-Barr Diet Plan and Sample Recipes

If you're on the Epstein-Barr diet, keep in mind that there are no rights or wrongs when it comes to selecting the recipes that will work best for you on a given day.

The following recipes are completely interchangeable, so you can follow these recipes any way you like. They are meant to be a guide to help you learn how to cook during your time on the diet, so you can build your confidence and become comfortable in the kitchen.

Arugula and Mushroom Salad

Ingredients:

- 5 oz. arugula washed
- 1 lb. fresh mushrooms
- 1/4 tsp. shoyu
- 1/2 red onion
- 1 tbsp. olive oil
- 1 tbsp. mirin
- For tofu cheese:
- 1/8 cup umeboshi vinegar
- 1/2 firm tofu

Instructions:

1. In a bowl, add the rinsed tofu. Crumble and pour in vinegar.
2. In a separate bowl add shoyu, red onions, salt, olive oil, and mirin. 3. Mix to combine.
3. Add in the arugula and toss to combine with the dressing.
4. Serve and enjoy.

Avocado, Cucumber, and Tomato Salad

Ingredients:

- 1/4 cup extra-virgin olive oil
- 1 pc. lemon, juiced
- 1/4 tsp. cumin, ground
- salt, to taste
- freshly ground black pepper, to taste
- 3 medium avocados, cubed
- 1-pint cherry tomatoes, halved
- 1 small cucumber, sliced into half-moons
- 1/3 cup corn
- 2 tbsp. cilantro, chopped

Instructions:

1. Combine avocados, cilantro, corn, cucumber, jalapeño, and tomatoes in a large bowl.
2. In a separate small container, whisk together lemon juice, cumin, and oil to make the salad dressing.
3. Season the dressing with salt and pepper.
4. Toss the salad gently while adding the dressing.
5. Serve immediately.

Chicken Salad

Ingredients:

- 1 small can of premium chunk chicken breast packed in water
- 1 stalk celery, large, finely chopped
- 1/4 cup reduced-fat mayonnaise
- 4 romaine leaves or red leaf lettuce, washed and trimmed
- 8 pcs. cherry tomatoes or 1 ripe tomato, quartered
- 1 cucumber, small and sliced thinly

Instructions:

1. Drain canned chicken and transfer to a bowl.
2. Put in celery and mayonnaise.
3. Mix lightly. Don't crush the chicken.
4. In a separate shallow bowl, place the lettuce neatly.
5. Add the chicken salad in the middle
6. Add tomatoes and cucumber slices to the plate.
7. Refrigerate before serving, cover with plastic wrap.

Egg Salad with Avocados

Ingredients:

- 3 medium-sized avocados
- 6 eggs, large and hard-boiled
- 1/3 red onion, medium size
- 3 celery ribs
- 4 tbsps. mayonnaise
- 2 tbsps. freshly squeezed lime juice
- 2 tsp. brown mustard
- 1/2 tsp. cumin powder
- 1 tsp. hot sauce
- salt
- pepper

Instructions:

1. Chop the eggs, celery, and onion.
2. Set aside the avocados, then combine the rest of the ingredients.
3. Slice the avocado in half to take out the pit.
4. Stuff the avocado by spooning the egg salad on its cave.
5. Serve and enjoy.

Vegetable Broth

Ingredients:

- 1 tbsp. oil
- 2 leeks, sliced
- 2 carrots, sliced
- 2 ribs celery
- 1/4 tsp. salt
- 8 cups water
- To make the soup:
- 1 tbsp. oil
- 2 cups potatoes, diced
- 1 cup mushrooms, diced
- 1-1/2 cups cauliflower, diced
- 1 cup onion, diced
- 1 cup celery, diced
- 1 cup carrot, diced
- 1-1/2 cups red beans, cooked
- 2 sprigs rosemary
- 4 sprigs thyme
- 2 cups spinach

Instructions:

1. To a pot on medium heat, add oil and leeks.
2. Cook for about three minutes or until they start to soften up.
3. Add carrots and top a few celery stalks with leaves.

4. Cover with water.
5. Add salt. Bring to a simmer and cook until carrots are very tender but not mushy.
6. Turn off the heat and let it cool down a little.
7. When the broth has cooled down, strain out the veggies.
8. Remove carrots and set them aside.
9. Squeeze most of the liquid out of the leeks and celery.

To cook the soup:

10. Add carrots to some of the broth and blend.
11. With a pot on medium heat, add oil, onions, raw carrots, and celery. Cook until onions are translucent, approximately 3 to 5 minutes.
12. Add broth, potatoes, and herbs.
13. Bring to a simmer and cook for 10 minutes.
14. Add cauliflower and red beans.
15. Simmer for another 5 minutes.
16. Add the package of frozen green beans and cook until the potatoes and cauliflower are tender, approximately for another 5 minutes.
17. At the end of cooking, add spinach.
18. Serve warm.

Apricot-Glazed Salmon

Ingredients:

- 1-1/3 pounds wild salmon filets
- 1/4 tsp. of crushed black pepper*
- 1 tbsp. virgin olive oil
- 1/2 cup of sodium-free vegetable broth
- 1 tbsp. Dijon mustard
- 1/3 cup of 100% apricot fruit spread
- 1 tsp. minced garlic

Instructions:

1. Preheat the grill over medium heat.
2. Pat salmon dry with a paper towel and cut it into four slices.
3. Season the skinless side with black pepper.
4. Wrap each piece with aluminum foil, with the skin side down. Fold the foil around the salmon securely to prevent oil from leaking.
5. In a bowl, combine the remaining ingredients.
6. Pour the mixture over the salmon slices.
7. Grill salmon for ten minutes.
8. Once cooked, allow the grilled filet to cool down before unwrapping.
9. Plate nicely and garnish with your favorite herbs before serving.

*black pepper may be substituted with white pepper

Salmon Salad

Ingredients:

- 2 large filets of wild salmon, either poached or grilled and then chilled
- 1 cup cherry tomatoes, halved
- 2 red onions, sliced
- 1 tbsp. balsamic vinegar
- 1 tbsp. capers
- 1 tbsp. fresh dill, finely chopped
- 1 tbsp. extra-virgin olive oil
- 1/4 tsp. pepper, freshly ground
- salt

Instructions:

1. Remove skin and bones from the cooled salmon.
2. Break salmon into chunks, and place them into a bowl.
3. Add tomatoes, red onion, and capers. Toss ingredients.
4. Combine balsamic vinegar, olive oil, and dill in a separate bowl.
5. Pour the mixture over the salmon chunks. Toss again.
6. Sprinkle it with salt and pepper to taste.
7. Chill salad for at least half an hour before serving.

Salmon with Avocados and Brussels Sprouts

Ingredients:

- 2 lbs. of salmon filet, divided into 4 pieces
- 1 tsp. ground cumin
- 1 tsp. onion powder
- 1 tsp. paprika powder
- 1/2 tsp. garlic powder
- 1 tsp. chili powder
- Himalayan sea salt
- black pepper, freshly ground

Avocado sauce:

- 2 chopped avocados
- 1 lime, squeezed for the juice
- 1 tbsp. extra-virgin olive oil
- 1 tbsp. fresh minced cilantro
- 1 diced small red onion
- 1 minced garlic clove
- Himalayan sea salt to taste
- black pepper, freshly ground

Brussels sprouts:

- 3 lbs. of Brussels sprouts
- 1/2 cup raw honey
- 1/2 cup balsamic vinegar
- 1/2 cup melted coconut oil

- 1 cup dried cranberries
- Himalayan sea salt
- black pepper, freshly ground

Instructions:

To make the salmon and avocado sauce:

1. Combine cumin, onion, chili powder, garlic, and paprika seasoned with salt and pepper. Mix well before dry rubbing on the salmon.
2. Place the salmon in the fridge for 30 minutes.
3. Preheat the grill.
4. In a bowl, mash avocado until the texture becomes smooth. Pour in all the remaining ingredients and mix thoroughly.
5. Grill salmon for 5 minutes on each side or until cooked.
6. Drizzle avocado on cooked salmon.

To prepare the Brussels sprouts:

1. Preheat the oven to 375°F.
2. Mix Brussels sprouts with coconut oil. Season with salt and pepper.

3. Place vegetables on a baking sheet and roast for about 30 minutes.
4. In a separate pan, combine vinegar and honey.
5. Simmer in slow heat until it boils and thickens.
6. Drizzle them on top of the Brussels sprouts.
7. Serve with the salmon.

Blueberry-Banana Overnight Oats

Ingredients:

- 1/2 cup old-fashioned oats
- 1/2 cup coconut milk, unsweetened
- 1/2 cup chia seeds, optional
- 1 tsp. maple syrup
- half piece of banana, mashed
- 1/2 cup blueberries
- a pinch of salt
- Optional: 1 tbsp. unsweetened flaked coconut

Instructions:

1. In a pint-sized jar, mix the oats, coconut milk, chia seeds, banana, maple syrup, and salt.
2. Top it with flaked coconut and fresh blueberries.
3. Cover it and leave it in a refrigerator overnight.

Salmon Soup

Ingredients:

- 1-3/4 cup coconut milk
- 2 tsp. dried thyme leaves
- 4 leeks, trimmed and sliced into crescents
- 6 cups seafood stock or chicken broth
- salt, for seasoning
- 3 cloves garlic, minced
- 1 lb. salmon, cut into bite-sized pieces
- 2 tbsp. avocado oil

Instructions:

1. Place avocado oil in a large saucepan or Dutch oven at low-medium heat. Add garlic and leeks.
2. Cook vegetables until slightly softened.
3. Pour in chicken or fish stock. Add in thyme and allow the mixture to simmer for approximately 15 minutes.
4. Season with salt to taste.
5. Add both coconut milk and salmon.
6. Bring the mixture up to a gentle simmer.
7. Cook until the fish is tender and opaque, then serve while hot.

Salad Medley

Ingredients:

- 4 artichokes, halved
- 1/2 avocado, sliced into thin wedges
- 1/2 red, yellow, or green bell pepper, thinly sliced
- 1/4 squash, thinly sliced
- 1/2 zucchini, thinly sliced
- 1/2 red, yellow, or green onion, thinly sliced
- 1 cup mushrooms, thinly sliced
- 1 cup broccoli
- 1/4 cup broccoli sprouts
- 1 cup cauliflower
- 1 cup spinach
- 1 cup kale
- 1 bunch leeks, chopped
- 1/4 cup raw sunflower seeds, sprouted
- 1/4 cup raw almonds, sprouted
- 1/4 cup garbanzo beans, sprouted
- 1/4 cup mung beans, sprouted
- 1/4 cup red or green lentils, sprouted
- 1/4 cup purple cabbage, shredded
- 2 tbsp. extra-virgin olive oil

Instructions:

1. Steam vegetables in a saucepan with 1-inch water for 5 to 10 minutes.
2. Transfer steamed vegetables into a serving bowl.
3. Drizzle with extra-virgin olive oil.
4. Toss the vegetables.
5. Serve immediately.

Conclusion

Thank you for taking the time to read this guide on managing Epstein-Barr Virus (EBV). Understanding this complex virus can be overwhelming, but by learning about its stages, symptoms, and natural ways to manage it, you've taken an important step toward reclaiming your health.

Coping with EBV isn't easy, but it's encouraging to know that you have options. By making positive changes in your diet, incorporating calming herbs, and replenishing your body with the right supplements, you can give your immune system the support it needs to fight back. Each choice you make—whether it's choosing a nutrient-packed meal, staying hydrated, or getting restorative sleep—helps create a stronger foundation for healing.

Remember, progress with EBV takes patience. Some days will feel better than others, and that's okay. Focus on the small victories, like increased energy or a reduction in symptoms, and celebrate those moments. Healing isn't about being perfect; it's about consistent care and kindness toward yourself.

You're not alone in this journey. EBV may present challenges, but it doesn't define you. Keep exploring what works best for you, and don't hesitate to seek support from loved ones or healthcare professionals. Whether it's adding a relaxation routine, trying a new recipe, or taking time to rest, every effort you make counts.

You have the power to take control of your well-being. By continuing to prioritize your health and staying informed, you're already on the path to feeling better. Thank you again for reading—you've got this! With time, care, and the steps outlined in this guide, brighter and healthier days are ahead. Take it one step at a time, and always trust in your ability to heal.

FAQs

Can EBV affect fertility or pregnancy?

EBV typically doesn't cause infertility or pregnancy complications, but severe symptoms can indirectly affect conception or pregnancy. Managing reactivations with care, stress reduction, and good nutrition is essential. Pregnant individuals should consult their healthcare provider for proper monitoring and management.

How can I prevent EBV reactivation during periods of stress?

Manage stress with mindfulness, deep breathing, or yoga. Prioritize 7–9 hours of sleep to support immunity. Eat a nutrient-rich diet, stay active, and consider supplements like zinc and ashwagandha. Set boundaries to avoid burnout and make time for relaxing activities.

Are there specific diets to follow alongside EBV if I have other conditions like diabetes or celiac disease?

Yes! Managing EBV while adhering to dietary needs for other conditions requires careful planning.

- ***For Diabetes:*** Focus on a low-glycemic, anti-inflammatory diet with lean proteins, non-starchy vegetables, and healthy fats. Avoid processed sugars and refined carbs, which can weaken your immune system.
- ***For Celiac Disease:*** Stick to a strict gluten-free diet while ensuring you get anti-inflammatory nutrients like omega-3s (via fish or seeds) and fiber from gluten-free grains like quinoa or brown rice.

Always consult with a dietitian or nutritionist to create a meal plan that meets your specific requirements while supporting EBV recovery and overall health.

Is EBV contagious during reactivation?

Yes, EBV can be mildly contagious during reactivation, though less so than the initial infection. It spreads mainly through saliva, so avoid sharing utensils, drinks, or kissing during an active phase. Most adults have already been exposed to EBV, so transmission risk often depends on individual immunity.

What are the long-term effects of EBV?

EBV can remain dormant and reactivate in some people, causing symptoms like fatigue or brain fog. Long-term effects are rare but more likely in those with weak immune systems or coexisting conditions. Proactive stress management, diet, and immune support can help minimize impacts.

Can children develop chronic EBV symptoms?

EBV is common in children and usually causes mild symptoms, but chronic EBV or post-viral fatigue is rare. Persistent symptoms like fatigue or swollen glands should be evaluated by a pediatrician. A nutrient-rich diet, rest, and reduced stress can help prevent complications.

References and Helpful Links

Medium, M. (2019, September 22). 12 foods that help fight Epstein-Barr Virus. Medical Medium. https://www.medicalmedium.com/blog/12-foods-that-help-heal-epstein-barr-virus

Rider, E. (2023, May 4). My Epstein-Barr Natural Treatment & healing protocol. Elizabeth Rider - Modern Healthy Living. https://www.elizabethrider.com/my-epstein-barr-treatment-natural-healing-protocol/

Facoep, J. P. C. D. (2022, October 13). Epstein-Barr virus: Symptoms, causes, treatment & prognosis. eMedicineHealth. https://www.emedicinehealth.com/epstein-barr_virus_infection/article_em.htm

Maria. (2021, November 16). EPSTEIN-BARR VIRUS – symptoms, causes, 10 ways to fight Epstein-Barr virus naturally and Epstein-Barr Diet – 24 healing foods. Ecosh. https://ecosh.com/epstein-barr-virus-symptoms-causes-10-ways-to-treat-epstein-barr-virus-naturally-and-epstein-barr-diet-24-healing-foods/Narayana Health. (n.d.). Narayana Health. https://www.narayanahealth.org/blog/mononucleosis-stages-symptoms-and-causes

Druckenmiller, R. (2021, August 12). How I Recovered from Epstein-Barr Virus (EBV) · Rachel's Nourishing Kitchen. Rachel's

Nourishing Kitchen. https://rachelsnourishingkitchen.com/healing-epstein-barr-ebv/

Hawkins, J. B., Delgado-Eckert, E., Thorley-Lawson, D. A., & Shapiro, M. (2013). The Cycle of EBV Infection Explains Persistence, the Sizes of the Infected Cell Populations and Which Come under CTL Regulation. PLoS Pathogens, 9(10), e1003685. https://doi.org/10.1371/journal.ppat.1003685

Kawada, J., Ito, Y., Ohshima, K., Yamada, M., Kataoka, S., Muramatsu, H., Sawada, A., Wada, T., Imadome, K., Arai, A., Iwatsuki, K., Ohga, S., & Kimura, H. (2023). Updated guidelines for chronic active Epstein–Barr virus disease. International Journal of Hematology, 118(5), 568–576. https://doi.org/10.1007/s12185-023-03660-5

UpToDate. (n.d.). UpToDate. https://www.uptodate.com/contents/clinical-manifestations-and-treatment-of-epstein-barr-virus-infection

www.ingramcontent.com/pod-product-compliance
Lightning Source LLC
LaVergne TN
LVHW012029060526
838201LV00061B/4532